How Not to Kill the Woman You Love

Your Guide to Surviving Her Menopause

How Not to Kill the Woman You Love

Your Guide to Surviving Her Menopause

Nina Hansen Machotka

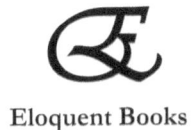

Eloquent Books

Eloquent Books
An imprint of Strategic Book Group
P.O. Box 333
Durham CT 06422
www.StrategicBookGroup.com

ISBN: 978-1-60911-307-0

Printed in the United States of America

Book Design: Stacie Tingen

To my mom
Now I get it

Table of Contents

To Talk or Not to Talk

After marriage and menstruation, menopause is the least talked about M word in the English language. Our grandmothers and mothers *never* talked about it, and if there was the occasional mention of "the change of life" by a father or uncle, it was accompanied with eyes rolling heavenwards. And what do you husbands, partners, relatives, sons and daughters talk about in secret?

Do you have a code for letting each other know the mood of the day, or if it's safe to come home, or if you should consider the "me" in the "it's the dog or me" threat that she issues daily? How do you avoid getting your heads cut off by the menopausal woman in your life? Surely, you've created a number of coping strategies. But because no one really talks about menopause, no one talks about concrete ways for you all to survive her change of life and not kill the woman you love.

Well, guess what? We are the baby-boomers, and we talk about everything! Now that we are in menopause and post-menopause, we'll talk about it from here to Sunday. But we also need to talk about some practical advice for all of you husbands, partners, kids, and animals on how to survive this incredibly complicated condition without mayhem, murder, or suicide—yours or hers.

A Small Intro to Your Guide

The books, journal articles, and online information I've researched on menopause are full of great facts and information about menopause for the menopausal woman. But there's virtually nothing for the spouses, partners, family, or animals. The scientific and medical books describe perimenopause and menopause as the "transitional phase" and the "change of life" phase with that high school textbook tone that we all know and love. (Personally, I describe these two as the "transitional phase between normal life and hell" and "welcome to hell" conditions.) Many of these books explain that certain symptoms may or may not occur (that's helpful), list available medicines or vitamins that *might* or *might not* lessen the symptoms (gee, thanks), and casually mention that depression or memory loss, panic attacks or increased alcohol intake, or lack of sexual feelings are **not caused** by menopause. Oh yeah?

Then why are there a zillion women who: 1) have never been depressed before, and are now depressed during menopause, sometimes to the point of not being able to function; 2) have *never* forgotten a phone number or a birthday in their entire lives, and now they don't remember a conversation from the night before; 3) used to enjoy sex and look forward to those Victoria's Secret catalogs every week, and now could give a flying hoot about "what might come up during the night;" 4) are suddenly gripped by fear, nausea, and difficulty breathing upon entering the local mall, their *favorite* place to hang out and shop for years?[1]

Further research led me to the "feel-good" books on menopause. You know the ones I mean—on and on about how menopause

---

1   One group takes these symptoms seriously as menopausal symptoms — the wonderful women at Project AWARE, the Association of Women for the Advancement of Research and Education (www.project-AWARE.org). I thank them for openly defying much of the medical world and publishing a myriad of menopausal symptoms and other enlightening information.

is the greatest experience of a woman's life, a huge source of creative energy, sexual passion, inspiration, and positive, forward thinking. I wanted to throw up. All I felt was anger and guilt for cursing the fact that I was waking up for the umpteenth time during the night, drenched in sweat, and throwing off the covers, sending the cat flying off the bed.

I concluded from my research that not only is the available information lacking in some truths for menopausal women, but there are absolutely no useful survival guides for the spouses, children, family members, and animals of the menopausal woman. This event is happening to all of you as well, yet no one's paying attention to you and your needs, least of all the menopausal woman, because she doesn't give a dang about your feelings, opinions, needs, or problems anymore (symptom number one).

So, this little book is written especially for you. For some background information, I briefly describe the physical, emotional, and psychological menopausal symptoms (all of which are *caused* by menopause in my mind, otherwise they wouldn't be called menopausal symptoms). Then I launch into the heart of the book for you—coping strategies in **10 easy steps**.

I recommend reading the steps from start to finish because some of the later steps depend upon you mastering the earlier ones. Learn them well, and your life will be transformed— you'll never have to suffer the wrath of your menopausal woman again!

Putting Menopause into Context

"You used to be nicer than this," a friend's husband said to her one day. "That's right," she hissed. "That was *before…*"

"Look," another friend said to her husband, "it's either a midlife crisis or a Mercedes…you choose."

A psychiatrist friend of my husband's once said "Everything that happens to a woman happens before, during, or after her period." Smart man. However, he didn't know anyone in menopause at the time because when menopause hits, everything happens *all* the time, and you'd better not mess with her if you value your life.

The dictionary defines menopause as, "The cessation of menstruation, occurring usually between 45 and 55. From the Greek *mèn* (month) + pause." (American Heritage dictionary, Third Edition). Well, that explains it all. According to this definition, menstruation stops. What's the big deal, you ask. You've no doubt already discovered there's a bit more than this. Finding this definition lacking, I thought I'd try one of my own. Here goes:

"The change in a woman's life/body/ mind/spirit, which includes anger, depression, confusion, memory loss, hot flashes, night sweats, cessation of menstruation after many false endings, and which threatens to topple your world no matter what you do." From the Greek *mèn* + pause—take a pause from men?

To begin coping with a menopausal woman, you need to think of menopause in two ways. One, it is your unwelcome houseguest who has decided to stay *way* too long. You may want to strangle that person, but to survive the visit you learn avoidance behaviors (you suddenly need to clean the garage for the first time in 10 years), and coping skills (you relearn your times tables by silently repeating them during the endless dinners, all with a frozen smile on your face).

Two, this is one of *the* most underrated events in a woman's life, with the possible exception of the first time she gets her bikini-line hair removed at the salon.

A Little Background

Menopause sucks, as one popular book[2] says.

That's all the background you need. But in case you're interested in more details, I've included a brief summary of the physical, psychological, and emotional symptoms (research that I discussed daily in long phone conversations with my girlfriends. At least that's what I told my husband when he wondered why the phone was glued to my ear for months).

Just when we thought it was safe. That's when menopause strikes. In a typical woman's life, she has endured the following (on average) up to the time of menopause: 480 months of menstrual periods; nine months of each pregnancy; childbirth (perhaps once, maybe up to seven or eight times, with an average 18 hours of labor); 5,400 diaper changes for *each* child; one to two years of sleepless nights for

---

2   One of many books by Joanne Kimes with "sucks" in the title.

each child; 280,000 meals cooked *just right*; roughly 14,000 trips to the supermarket; more miles than 20 Indy-500s between school, soccer, music lessons, dance lessons, doctors, dentists, and college dorms; 25-30 years of Johnny Carson or Monday Night Football to keep her husband company; and 2,500 phone conversations with her mother-in-law (not her choice).

At some point in her late 40s, it all quiets down. She's sitting on the couch one night thinking, "Gee, the kids are nearly grown or out of the house and no longer resemble Martians. Her husband seems content with his job and hobbies, perhaps they could take up sailing or travel to an exotic island…" BLAM! The first hot flash hits.

Her entire body tingles with pinpricks down to her fingertips and toes. Her face is flushed, her scalp is prickly, and she starts to sweat. This is not the good sweat one feels after a workout at the gym or a jog around the block. This feels like Washington DC in August, except that it's the middle of January in Wisconsin. The sweat drips from her scalp, down her neck, front, and back. Even her shins are wet. It's like a niacin rush, burning hot from the *inside* out. She fans herself, paces around the room, pulls her clothes away from her skin, blows on her chest. She seriously considers stripping naked and standing on the porch in 10-degree weather. Screw the neighbors.

And then, it's over. She cools down, her breathing returns to normal, she's calm. That wasn't so bad. As long as they don't strike too often, she figures she can handle this. Then she starts to shiver. She is drenched, and the slightest movement of air feels like the thrust from a 747 jet engine. She runs to the dresser, pulls out a sweatshirt and sweatpants, and huddles next to the dog on the couch. Don't even think about seeing her in lingerie again.

After awhile, you both forget about it, continue your backgammon game, think about making love tonight. You climb into bed, turn towards her, and she yelps, "Don't touch me!"

"Why? What?" You wonder what the heck you've done.

The night sweats have arrived. They're different from hot flashes. Typically the first one starts about two minutes after she climbs into bed. Forget about making love. Night sweats sap energy and desire and leave her feeling just plain icky. Throughout the night, she wakes up and throws off the covers. Everything is drenched—pajamas, sheets, pillow case. Then the shivering starts, and the covers are yanked up again. This can occur two to five times a night. While you snore on.

Despite these roller-coaster symptoms, the first week is almost exciting. She's thinking, *Yeah! No more periods!* But the periods don't just stop. Oh no. They stop for a few months, then return on your first vacation, and of course she hasn't brought any supplies along because there was no need to. Then they stop for eight months. Then she gets another one. The goal is to reach one year without periods, then she is most likely "done." You get the picture—it ain't over till it's over.

The second week she starts taking sleeping pills. This is no longer exciting, this sucks. The third week she's pulling her hair out, reading everything she can get her hands on about relieving the symptoms. She's on the phone with her friends, doctors, her mom, her older sister who has been going through this for years. They all have the same advice: get used to it, it's not going away for a very long time.

"How long?" she asks (her husband secretly listening in on the extension in the next room).

"Months, years; could be the rest of your life," her sister informs her.

"Oh my god," she whispers. "After everything I've been through, I've gotta live with this the rest of my life?"

"Join the crowd, sweetie!" her sister laughs.

As she hangs up, she hears a strange crumpling sound, as if someone in the other room has collapsed onto the floor.

After a couple of months, she's resigned. Otherwise, she'll go stark-raving mad (not to mention what *you're* going through, but we'll get to that). Unfortunately and seriously, many women do go mad. According to too many experts, the connections are "fuzzy" between menopause and increased alcoholism, depression, memory loss, panic attacks, hives, migraines, and so on. My question again is why do so many women have nervous breakdowns around 50, or become alcoholics, or fall into serious depressions? The facts are staring us in the face—we know them, you know them, why don't the experts know them?

After a year, she's ready to commit hara-kiri. And you're ready to be her second. (Read about the ritual of Seppuku, and you'll understand this role.)

One of the ways you can help her get through her hot flashes—and therefore help yourself so you can get a decent meal or make love again—is with some humor (but not too much! This is a delicate procedure.) My husband, bless his soul, calls them my "noble moments." If I can't get outside for fresh air, I have to sit absolutely still, head held high, arms extended out from my body, and let the sweat roll.

I once saw a bumper sticker that said, "They're not hot flashes, they're power surges!"

Be creative. I bet you'll come up with some good phrases or terms that will help lighten these prickly moments.

Enter, the Body Snatchers

What happens to a woman's body when she's going through menopause? As menopause begins, the ovaries start changing and hormones go crazy—too much of one, not enough of another, and everything gets thrown out of balance. Periods become incredibly heavy, then sporadic. They stop for a few months, then return. They stop again. This cycle can continue for two to three years. Some women are lucky—their periods stop one day and they're done. In my unofficial research, these women are rare.

Once the ovaries stop their egg production, the hormone *estrogen* all but disappears. Estrogen is *the* power hormone in a woman's body. It circulates through the body and drives the functions of the hypothalamus in the brain. Now, the hypothalamus is a marvelous part of the brain that moderates a ton of stuff and keeps things from going haywire.

Here are a few of the body functions it moderates:

- cravings, hunger and salt, feeding reflexes

- thirst and water preservation

- testicular and ovarian functions

- metabolism

- blood pressure regulation and heart rate

- mood and behavioral functions

- balance

- sleep cycles

- body temperature

- bladder function

- energy levels

No wonder women crave salted peanuts, bump into walls, race for the bathroom, sweat one minute, shiver the next, and are irritable 23 hours a day. Once you realize the importance of this gland, weight gain, aching joints, vaginal dryness, migraines, and memory loss are no surprise. It's a miracle most women continue functioning against these odds.

There are ways to combat these symptoms, hormone-replacement therapy being one of them, but that has major drawbacks. To keep this guide simple, I suggest "Googling" these topics on the Internet; you'll find thousands of pages that offer many choices.

Women on the Verge

What happens to a woman psychologically and emotionally during menopause? Apart from the obvious fact that those body snatchers have swept away the kind, gentle, loving woman you fell in love with, married, raised children with, shared more than half a lifetime with, and have now replaced her with Medusa, snakes and knives at the ready? A lot.

This is the scary stuff, for both of you. Scary for her because she cannot control what is happening. Scary for you because no matter what you do, it'll be wrong. You need to know that these will probably disappear, and you'll resume a normal life...if you can hang in there long enough. Here are some common symptoms, which you already know all too well:

- Extreme, prolonged anger, the likes of which neither you nor she has ever seen

- Depression, dread, anxiety, and a ton of tears

- Declining interest in hobbies, exercise, those "feel good" things she used to do

- Self-esteem hits rock bottom; she feels absolutely worthless

- Husband's and children's problems become laughable

- Paranoid feelings and conspiracy theories arise (for example, she's convinced the dog has learned to open the frig and steal things—she KNOWS she bought a chicken the day before, but where the heck is it?)

- Having sex seems like jump-roping at this age—what's the point?

- General dislike of any woman under 30, especially anyone who looks like Halle Barry, Angelina, or the frigging Playboy twins

- Newly acquired love of grappa, brandy, vodka, tequila, box wine—any liquid that numbs the emotional roller coaster or makes her husband more interesting as the evenings drag on.

Depression and anxiety top the list for most women. Depression takes different forms. It can be subtle—sleeping more, not wanting to go out in the evenings, letting the bills pile up, more frozen dinners, gaining some weight, not wanting sex. It can be debilitating—gaining a lot of weight, prolonged crying spells, failing tasks at work, not caring about the kids or you or the dog, drinking a lot more, not wanting sex. It can be devastating—alcoholism serious enough for intervention and treatment, nervous breakdown, suicide or murder, not wanting sex.

Anxiety takes on various forms as well. There's a general feeling of something bad about to happen, or not being able to shake off the feeling that something bad *has* happened to the kids or you. Planning meals and having people over for dinner is a nightmare—anxious confusion of what to cook, where to start, the timing of the different dishes, how to get it all to the table without dropping anything. She's overwhelmed and *knows* she's going to fail and disappoint everyone. I have found myself walking back and forth in the kitchen for 20 minutes, going from drawer to frig to oven to cabinets to counter-tops, and…nothing. Not one plate out, not one fork or spoon, food spread out and still packaged.

And what are you going through while your menopausal woman is walking in circles? Probably some depression, anxiousness, and confusion yourself.

If you're going to survive this phase of life, you've got to pull yourself together and start practicing the 10 steps outlined for you in the next chapter. I know it would be much easier to stay late at the office every night, or drink that third beer to wash it all away. But in the end, those behaviors don't help anyone, especially you. They gloss over the reality and don't give you any specific skill sets to adapt, cope, and survive.

Buck up and read on! You're about to learn some secrets that no one has ever bothered to teach you. Courage!

Your 10 Steps
to Blissful Peace

Now you know the symptoms. It's time to learn the skills that will help you adapt, cope, and survive. Here we go.

Step 1. Think terrible twos

Remember the terrible twos your children went through? Good. First and foremost, think of the menopausal woman in your life as the adult version of the terrible twos. It may take the form of blackmail (my friend who demanded the Mercedes or else), or the ultimate attention getter (throwing a major tantrum, preferably in a quiet, posh restaurant), or the harshest resort to get one's way (threatening to withhold sex forever).

She feels no one is listening to her or paying attention until she throws that tantrum. Communication is a weird code that makes sense to everyone *else* in the room. Those wonderful little tasks like buying all the right ingredients for dinner are overwhelming. And who gives a flying leap about dinner anyway? Fix it yourself. And why shouldn't she wear one purple sock and one red one? Two year olds dance in the middle of the living room when company is over. Is there a problem?

Step 2. Learn to become invisible

This is one of the most important steps. Learn this one well and you'll be on your way to peaceful bliss.

Becoming invisible is necessary when you want to get out of the house but can't. This step applies to spouses or partners, teenagers, in-laws, and the dog. (**Note**: Cats don't have to worry about this step, they've been masters at it for centuries. If you can find your cat, ask her how she does it.)

It takes a little practice to look like the standing lamp in the corner of the living room. This trick is useful when your mom and wife are discussing men and they want you to stick around, join in, voice your opinion (an invitation I suggest you turn down).

It may take more practice to turn the same shade of mustard as your refrigerator, but this is a particularly smart transformation when you find yourself stuck in the kitchen while she's making gravy for the Thanksgiving turkey or trying to get the soufflé to rise.

As time goes on, and you "disappear" more and more, you'll notice your menopausal woman relaxing, becoming happy or giddy at times. It's not that she doesn't like having you in the house, you understand, it's just that she doesn't like having you in the house. Be patient, this will change.

Step 3. Take up sports

This helps in a number of ways. You get some exercise to work off that gut you've been nurturing for the last 20 years. You get to have a guy-thing experience, and you can hit the ball (or your buddies) with all the ferocity and anger building up inside you living with your Medusa. But most important, it gets you *out of the house* and you don't have to keep practicing your broom closet imitation.

Step 4. Become a yes-person

It's really simple. Y-E-S. Try it again. Y-E-S. Practice in front of the bathroom mirror every morning. Once you've perfected the pronunciation, apply it to *everything* she says. Want to take out the garbage? YES! Want to go to the Smith's tonight for bridge? YES! Want to clean your room? YES! Shall we make tofu burgers with chicken livers for dinner tonight? YES! You want to have sex? Uh…watch out for that one and read **Step 8**.

My mother once told us she had found the secret of life.

"The secret of life," she said, "is that if you all just do things *my* way everyone will be happy!" Mind those words during this phase of her life and just say YES!

Step 5. Learn to cook

Cooking can actually be fun and rewarding! Why else do you think she's done it all these years, hmmmm? You get to think up something new every night so you don't have to hear from the kids, "we're having *that* again?" You get to hone your planning skills, your organizational skills, your diplomatic skills when the family wants five different dishes to satisfy each food preference. You certainly get to know the joys of preparing food for two to three hours and then watching it all disappear, without a word from anyone, in 10 minutes flat.

After you learn to cook, learn to clean up! Cleaning up the kitchen after meals is an inspirational experience. You won't need an after dinner drink, you won't need the ballgame or the sitcom, you won't even need to sit and relax anymore! You'll find that staying in the kitchen alone, facing five sets of dinner and dessert plates, twenty-five sets of glasses, knives, forks, and spoons, three serving dishes, four pots and three pans, is simply marvelous. The potential for self-actualization at that moment is awesome. Why else do you think she's done it all these years?

Step 6. Switch the radio station to '70s rock

There is no time like the past. This is particularly useful for you teenagers. Who needs Rihanna when you can have "I Wanna Rock With You All Night" (very early Michael Jackson), "Keep the Fire Burning" (Loggins & Messina), "Down to You" (Joni Mitchell) or "Your Song" (Elton John). But wait, just when you think you've stomached enough '70s *soft* rock, the Doobie Brothers will come blasting on with "Long Train Runnin'", undoubtedly one of the best tunes ever. She'll be rocking out, dancing in the living room. And you know what? That woman can dance. Keep your mouths shut and let her dance. The last thing she needs to hear is "Ew, Daaaad, Mommy's dancing! It's weird!"

This is a good time for **Step 2** for you, kid. This is *her* music from *her* era when *she* was on top of the world (as you think you are right now).

Step 7. Become an interesting conversationalist

First things first: Read **Step 4**. That technique is still the most effective for these "philosophy of life" discussions after some wine has been consumed. However, you may be called upon to participate in the conversation, to be more present, so here are some practical stock phrases and answers:

"I hear ya, yeah, that's interesting."

"I didn't know that!"

"You think so? I *never* thought of it that way."

"Tell me more."

"Don't stop, I'm listening! It's fascinating!"

After awhile, you can think up some of your own to better fit your personal style and character.

Step 8. Sex

Notice the title. It's not "Have More Sex" or "Don't Have Sex" or "Be More Sexy" or "Sex, Honey?" It's just "Sex." And it's a ticking bomb.

This is probably the most touchy area while living with your Medusa. You need to understand that to a menopausal woman, the thought of sex seems as useful as a car without wheels. A friend who was in the middle of menopause told me that she finally understood the "bimbo" factor and considered encouraging her husband to go find one.

Don't try to explain that it's fun, or that it feels good, or that it brings you closer together, or that you still desire her, or that you just need it, because she will look at you and seriously wonder how she ever married you.

But don't despair! Things *do* get better. Especially once the periods finally stop for good. She'll realize this is a pretty good place to be in...no more fuss, no more muss, no more planning trips around her periods, no more worry (as in not the remotest chance of getting pregnant). Maybe sex IS a good thing. But watch out, once that thought re-enters her head, she may not be looking at you when she thinks it. Especially if you're still wearing that torn flannel shirt every night. Or those really attractive sweat pants that don't hide enough of your stomach, which in turn now hides too much of...well, you know.

Maybe, just maybe, sex would be great again if you remember the days of your early romance. Listen, you guys have totally forgotten how to ride a bike and how to go about getting sex (and making it interesting). Which is strange because you were experts at it by the time you were teenagers. Remember? All those beautiful, romantic, loving, and sexy words? "Oh baby, you have the most beautiful eyes." "Those lips, what cute ears, your hair is like water falling down your back, what a great neck you have, you look SO sexy in those jeans, they really turn me on, I love kissing you, tell me you love me forever..."

Is it coming back to you? Oh boy. You used every romantic trick in the book you could think of to get us to sleep with you, and guess what? Most of the time it worked! Lies, lies, lies, but who cared? It sounded great to us and we fell for it every time. Of course, we took it a bit more seriously than you did. I mean we really believed you and managed to get you to the alter!

There is a famous saying that sums up the difference between men and women when it comes to love and sex: Men use love to get sex, and women use sex to get love. Well, one little fact you need to know is she probably won't be using sex to get your love now. But! She still needs your love and affection, and once you give that to her freely, you'll be making love again.

Give it a try. A little mood music, a little fire in the fireplace, a little sweet talk, a little wine, a lot of back rubbing, and see how the night goes.

Step 9. Don't ask what she's doing or *why* she's doing it

She doesn't know, and this is a sure-fire way to start a fight. She hasn't asked you what you've been up to all these years in your so-called workshop. She hasn't asked why you're rebuilding your '72 VW engine for the eighth time. She certainly hasn't asked *why* you insist on barbequing the steaks to death every 4th of July while claiming to be the best cook on the block.

So, if you find the milk carton in the cupboard, don't ask why it's there. Put it in the frig, take the box of cereal out, and put that back in the cupboard. If you find her bras in your underwear drawer, admire them and put them back in her drawer. If you see a belly-button ring one day when she's undressing for bed, tell her it looks better than your daughter's does. And if you find her walking in circles in the kitchen and dinner is two hours late, don't ask what she's doing, join in and do a tango! And then apply **Step 5**.

Step 10. When all else fails...

After you've tried, and hopefully mastered, all the steps, if things are still rough, if your menopausal woman is still more Medusa than Venus, and you're getting to the end of your rope, here's what you do.

Go out and buy yourself a nifty little red sports car, preferably a convertible. Go cruise the boulevard with the other guys (pay no attention to how young they all look), and watch the foxy chicks go by. Park in front of the local nightclub and *believe* that you've still "got it." Believe that you are one handsome dude who can catch a 19-year-old honey-pie with the way you raise one eyebrow and smile that sexy smile. Don't worry, in the dim light no one will notice your false teeth.

Make sure you're spotted by your friends' children who are also hanging out at the club so that word will *be sure* to get right back to your Medusa that you are *out there, on the make, lookin' good, and you're getting some pretty hot responses! Whoa!*

When you get home, you won't believe the change in your Medusa. Believe me.

Do this last step just right, and you'll see the difference—because you will have given her **the** biggest belly-laugh of her entire life, and she will always, always love you for that.

* * * * * * *

Coming next: *Your Guide to Surviving Her Post-Menopause.*

Did something fall to the floor in the next room?